Selsabil DABOUSSI
Mariem CHAABANE
Samira MHAMDI

Lung ultrasound at the bedside

Selsabil DABOUSSI
Mariem CHAABANE
Samira MHAMDI

Lung ultrasound at the bedside

The clinician's stethoscope

Imprint
Any brand names and product names mentioned in this book are subject to trademark, brand or patent protection and are trademarks or registered trademarks of their respective holders. The use of brand names, product names, common names, trade names, product descriptions etc. even without a particular marking in this work is in no way to be construed to mean that such names may be regarded as unrestricted in respect of trademark and brand protection legislation and could thus be used by anyone.

Cover image: www.ingimage.com

This book is a translation from the original published under ISBN 978-620-3-45039-2.

Publisher:
Sciencia Scripts
is a trademark of
Dodo Books Indian Ocean Ltd. and OmniScriptum S.R.L publishing group

120 High Road, East Finchley, London, N2 9ED, United Kingdom
Str. Armeneasca 28/1, office 1, Chisinau MD-2012, Republic of Moldova, Europe
Printed at: see last page
ISBN: 978-620-5-75600-3

LUNG ULTRASOUND AT THE BEDSIDE: BASIC PRINCIPLES AND RELEVANCE TO THE CLINICIAN'S DAILY PRACTICE

PREAMBLE

Bedside ultrasound by the healthcare professional has revolutionized patient care worldwide, providing clinicians with immediate answers to clinical questions, and guiding procedures safely.This monograph represents a concise guide to thoracic ultrasound for any clinician who is involved in the management of a patient in a clinical setting and helps answer specific questions about diagnosis and common disease processes.A case study is integrated in this monograph allowing the adoption of pulmonary and pleuroparietal ultrasound, as an extension of the clinical examination, a means available at the patient's bed, non expensive and non irradiating, in the clinical reasoning of the patient.This monograph is dedicated to all specialties that manage a patient in a clinical setting: (pulmonology, internal medicine, emergency, resuscitation, cardiology)

Pulmonary ultrasound Why?

✓ **Benefits**

- Examination available at the patient's bedside

- For several pathologies, more sensitive and specific than conventional imaging

- Result of the examination obtained instantly

- Dynamic assessment (compared to standard chest X-ray / chest CT)
- Fast learning curve

- No ionizing radiation

✓ **Disadvantages**

- Only pathologies involving the diaphragm, chest wall, subpleural lung abnormalities, and pleura can be imaged ($\approx$70% of explorable pleura).

PLAN

I. INTRODUCTION AND BACKGROUND

In 1880, the Curie brothers discovered the piezoelectric effect producing ultrasound. Their first application was not medical, but military, with **the "hydrophone"**, ancestor of the **Sonar**, allowing the detection of submarines during the First World War.The use of ultrasound in medical diagnosis dates back to the late 1930s.

Karl Dussik, an Austrian physician, and his brother **Friederick Dussik**, a physicist, used ultrasound to visualize the anatomy of the brain and the presence of any tumors.Many consider **Dussik** to be the father of clinical ultrasound. The first ultrasound scanner was born in 1951, from the collaboration of two Englishmen, Dr. John Wild and the electronics engineer J. Reid.Since then, it has undergone continuous progress until today, particularly in terms of size and manageability, providing physicians with an easy-to-use tool at the patient's bedside. (1)In the following decades and during the Second World War, the technique was developed and named sonar (Sound Navigation And Ranging).

The principles and technologies leading to the development of sonar have also been noted among physicians.In the following years, the use of medical ultrasound was mainly developed and adopted in specialties such as **cardiology, radiology** and **obstetrics,**

but its use in most other specialties remained limited until the 1990s.

The pleuropulmonary ultrasound is said to be focal: it is integrated in the **extension of t h e interrogation and the clinical examination of the patient.**

It is a **targeted examination,** related to the suspected pathology.
It allows to confirm or refute possible diagnostic hypotheses by increasing the clinical sensitivity.This is not an exhaustive complementary examination that remains t h e prerogative of the radiologist or cardiologist.

It is sometimes referred to as a "clearance ultrasound", although the term clinical ultrasound seems more appropriate.It can be repeated if necessary according to changes in the patient's clinical condition.

This is why the ultrasound scanner is considered by some professionals and authors as **"the future stethoscope of the clinician".**

Numerous studies have demonstrated its interest in the management of patients in emergency situations, and especially in the era of COVID where patients cannot be moved because of their critical respiratory condition and fear of the risk of infection, this interest being of a diagnostic, therapeutic or orientation nature.

The indication and use of clinical ultrasound has become widespread for all specialties,According toBobbia et al. in a 2014 study of 50 French emergency departments, the use of clinical ultrasound is divided between 30% for echocardiography,14% for FAST(FocusedAssessmentwithSonographyforTrauma), 14% for urinary tract, 11% forpulmonary ultrasound, and 7% forvenous ultrasound of the lower extremities.

The remaining 24% are shared between biliary tract analysis, gynecology, soft tissues and osteoarticular. (6)

This does not mean that everything has to be examined by ultrasound, but that one has to know what is useful. For this purpose, evidence-based medicine should be used.It is a clinical ultrasound that must be integrated into a reasoning, within other clinical signs.It is important to know the sensitivity and specificity of the target images, in order to progress in a probabilistic reasoning.

It is important to understand the limitations of ultrasound and to know how to refer to the **"gold standard"** examination when necessary.

Currently, there is no evidence of benefit of clinical ultrasound in terms of morbidity and mortality. However, the gain in diagnostic efficiency leading to an adapted therapeutic prescription or orientation in emergency situations strongly suggests a benefit for the patient. The studies on the gain brought by ultrasound techniques clinical trials usually show that it is in situations of diagnostic uncertainty where this gain is major.

The history of lung ultrasound in brief

The use of lung ultrasound (LUS) for the evaluation of pulmonary diseases such as pleural effusion and pulmonary embolism has been known since the birth and early years of medical ultrasound.

Despite these early efforts, the use of LUS as a clinical tool has long been considered limited to the evaluation of pleural effusion.

This assumption was based on the fact **that the lungs** contain **air, which** makes it impossible to assess by ultrasound.

Initially, the use of the LUS as an assessment tool for horses with respiratory diseases challenged this dogma.

Norman W. Rantanen(1) reported the use of LUS for the evaluation and diagnosis of conditions such as **pulmonary consolidations, atelectasis, abscesses, pleural effusion, empyema and pneumothorax** in horses.

In addition, Rantanen's article contains descriptions of **vertical and horizontal reverberation artifacts** as well as **the concept of pleural blade movement during breathing** in **normal lungs**, and **its absence in pneumothorax**

• These signs and artifacts were later to be considered as **key concepts in LUS**.

• Subsequent work by **Daniel Lichtenstein** evaluating the use of LUS in humans led to the renaissance of LUS as an essential diagnostic modality in **the**

evaluation of patients with known or suspected chest disease.

• For this reason, Lichtenstein is considered by many to be the father of modern LUS. Among Lichtenstein's many works, particularly the use of LUS for the diagnosis of pneumothorax and interstitial syndrome (IS) (e.g., pulmonary edema, acute respiratory distress syndrome) in an intensive care unit are important.

Another milestone in lung ultrasound was the publication in 2012 of the first international evidence-based recommendations **for bedside lung ultrasound**

II. INTEREST OF PLEUROPULMONARY ULTRASOUND

This is one of the most studied fields of application of clinical ultrasound, notably through the work of Lichtenstein (20-22).He compared the diagnostic performance of auscultation, chest radiography and pleuropulmonary ultrasound in respiratory distress, proving undeniably the superiority of ultrasound in terms of sensitivity and specificity for the diagnosis of pleural effusion, alveolar condensation and interstitial syndrome (Appendix 2). **(Appendix 2)** The practice of clinical pleuropulmonary ultrasound applied in the context of dyspnea is also integrated into diagnostic algorithms, the most famous of which is the Blue Protocol **(Appendix 3).**

III. PRINCIPLES OF PULMONARY ULTRASOUND

A basic understanding of ultrasound is a prerequisite for performing clinical ultrasound

Ultrasound is an imaging technique that uses ultrasound. Ultrasound is sent through a probe transmitter into a defined area of the body. The different organs send back the ultrasounds to a receiver placed in the same probe. The recorded echoes, processed by a computer, show the obstacles encountered by the signal. The measurement of the amplitude makes it possible to distinguish a soft tissue (muscles) from a hard tissue (bones) and the measurement of the duration which separates the emission from the reception of each echo (duration of a round trip) makes it possible to determine the dimensions of the observed organs.

1. Physical Basics:

A wave can be defined as an oscillating disturbance of particles passing through a medium. A sound wave is an example of such an oscillating disturbance propagating through a medium. A sound wave is a mechanical wave and therefore requires a medium to carry the wave energy from one place to another. Different media can be used to propagate a sound wave (e.g. air, liquid). The propagation is done from near to near as a longitudinal wave. This means that the individual molecules of the medium only vibrate in the same direction as the sound waves. The wave "travels" by transferring the vibration through the molecules of the medium A sound wave works like a bat: a blind bat needs to form an image of its environment. It sends ultra-sounds which are not audible by the man superior to 15 khz. These sound waves will touch the objects and reflect back to the bat's brain, which will give it a precise map of its environment

What is an ultrasound?

Ultrasound travels through the air at the same speed as sound $v = 330$ m/s. Their frequencies are higher than those detected by the human ear, which only hears frequencies f such that 20 Hz $<$ f $<$ 20 kHz. The ultrasound is much higher between 1Mhz and 50 MHZ.

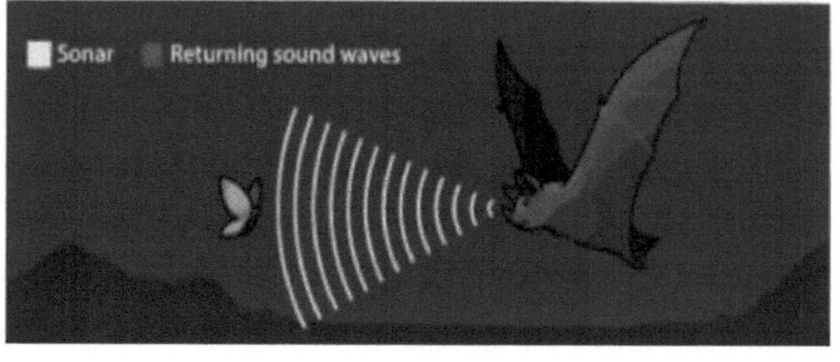

Figure 1: Echolocation. Image adapted from Arizona State University -Ask A Biologist

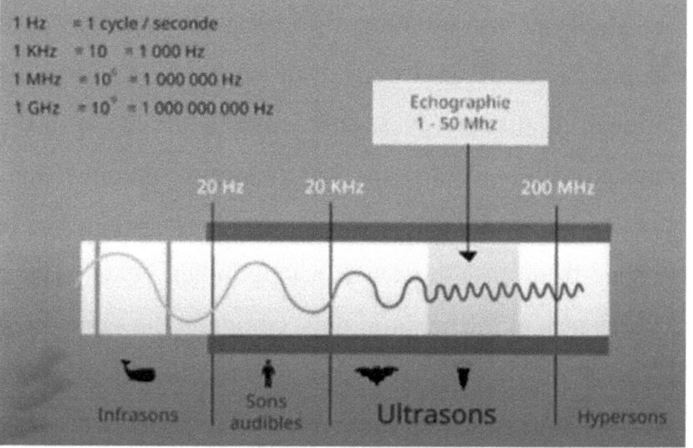

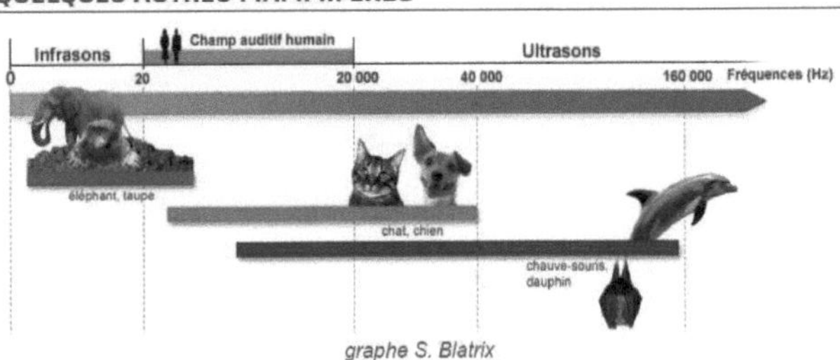

graphe S. Blatrix

The medical ultrasound uses a frequency of 1 to 20 MHz and works on this model to produce an ultra sound the probe emits an electric current. This electric current passes through the piezoelectric crystals which cause vibrations that result in the creation of ultra-sounds.The beam of ultra-sounds is going to meet objects, targets, which are going to entrain a reflection of these beams towards the probe which are thus the transmitter and the receiver and which are going to allow them to produce an image which is the image on the screen.

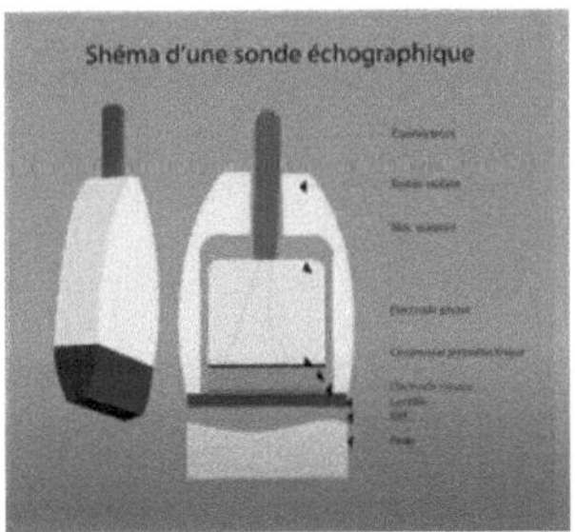

The sound wave is characterized by a length and an amplitude, it is longitudinal. The frequency is the number of cycles, that is to say the length of waves per second

1 cycle over one second = 1Hz

10 cycles per second = 10 HZ

The wave propagates by encountering an elastic and deformable material medium, which means that it cannot move in a vacuum, it needs a support, be it fabric, air or water.It will locally deform the tissue by causing oscillations of the molecules around their equilibrium position.To produce images, you need obstacles.

The beam will encounter two types of obstacles:

✓ The first type of obstacle: these are small targets, for example cells within the lung parenchyma, which will result in a granular image

✓ The second type is the interfaces: these are the limits that separate the organs and these limits will appear hyperechoic as a white line

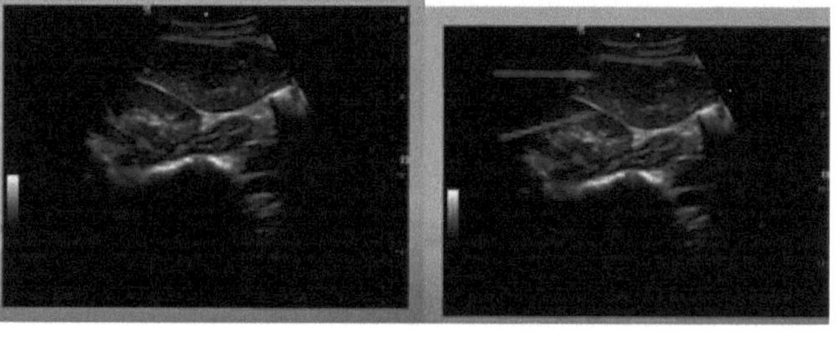

By hitting these obstacles, the wave undergoes different phenomena and the rays return to the probe which records them and emits an image on the screen.

Take home messages

□ Each fabric has its own resistance to US (depends on the density and speed of sound (elasticity))

□ Resistance= Acoustic impedance

□ The difference in Impedance between 2 media creates an Interface

□ The ultrasound wave is reflected on the interfaces and is at the origin of the ultrasound image

□ The intensity of the reflection of the US depends on the difference of impedances at the interface (air/water..)

In ultrasound, it is the interfaces, the boundaries between organs, that are the basis of the image as opposed to conventional radiology where we are more interested in the density of the organs

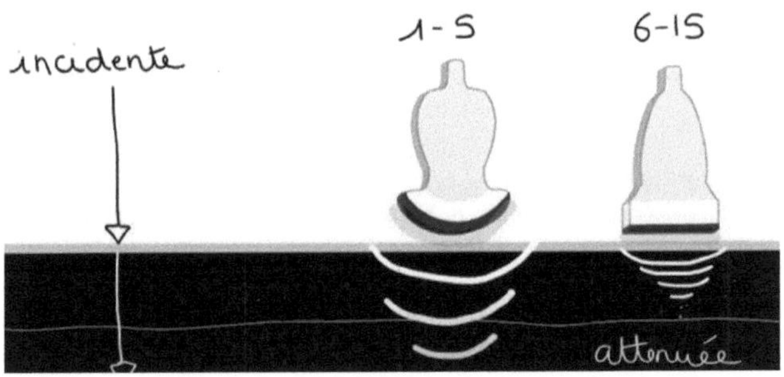

The probe emits an incident wave: this acoustic energy passes through the skin, the gel and then progressively through the different tissues towards the depth We say that the acoustic energy is transmitted, it allows to obtain the images located in depth

However the beam will lose energy
✓ Either because the Energy will be dispersed

✓ Either because the Energy is going to be deviated by several phenomena*
and we say that the Energy is attenuated with an exponential decrease
The frequency will also have an important effect on the attenuation in fact the more the frequency increases and the more the energy is attenuated by Diffusion and Absorption Hence a poor depth display for high frequencies

Take home messages
☐ Highest frequencies: linear probes can only be used for surface structures
☐ Low frequencies: convex probes are used for deep structures

***The phenomena undergone by the wave**

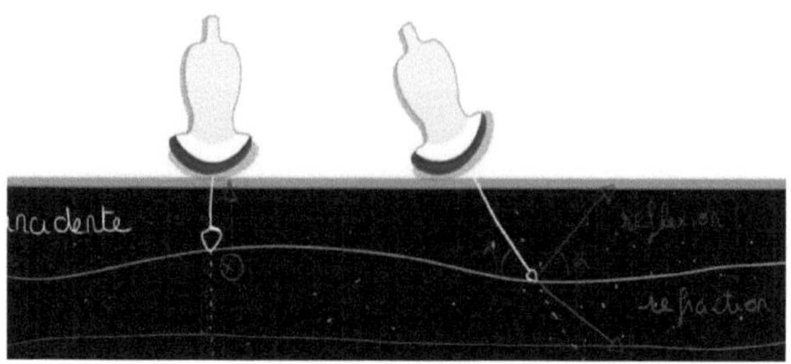

✓ **The reflection**

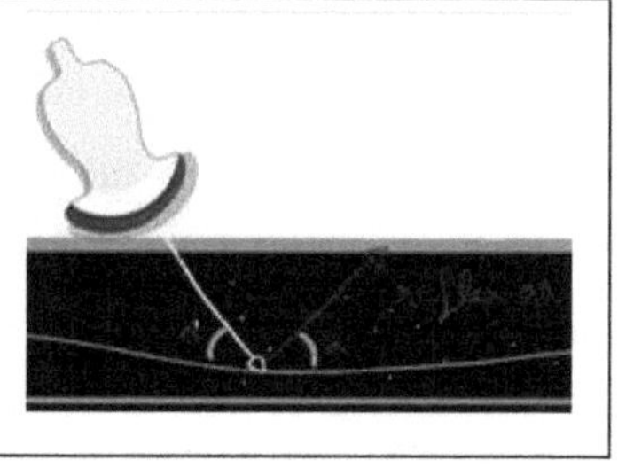

Return of the beam with an angle equivalent to the incident wave

✓ **Refraction**

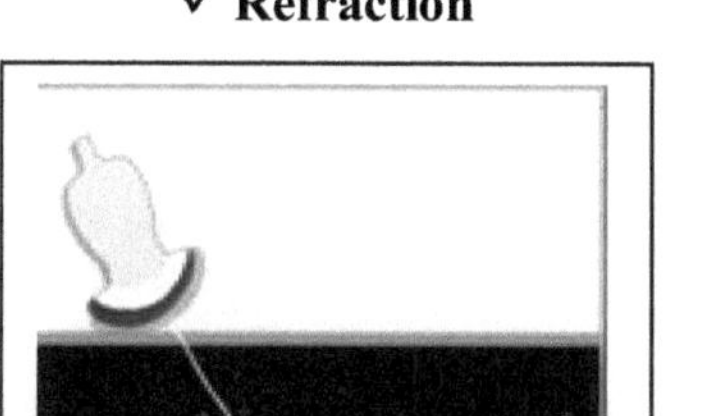

When the wave passes from one medium to another with different speeds the wave is deflected Unless the incident wave arrives perfectly perpendicular to the interface in which case there is no refraction

When it arrives on a small target this wave undergoes scattering and diffraction. Indeed a cell of small size compared to the length of the wave is reflective and generates waves in all directions around it also called interference noise or spicule the granite or grain of the parenchyma.

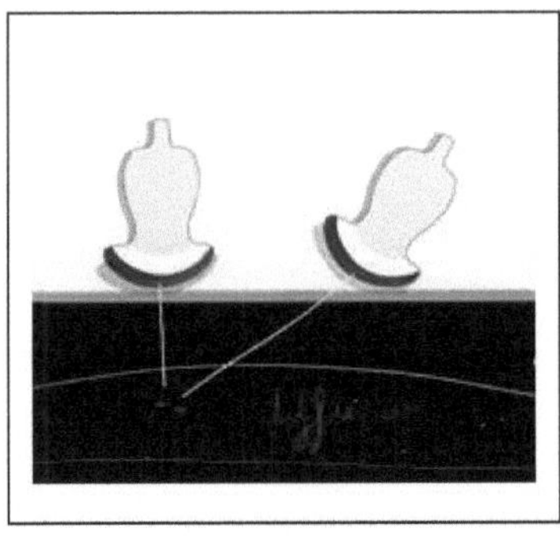

Whatever the incidence of the wave that arrives on the parenchyma, the diffusion is the same, so the image of the parenchyma is identical, whatever the way in which the probe was placed on the patient.

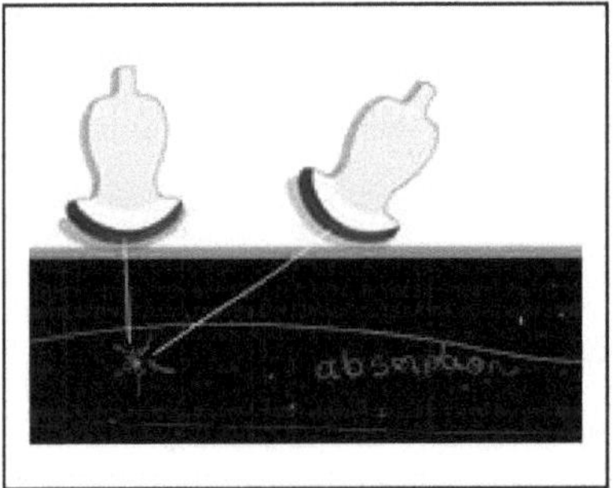

The waves can be absorbed by the fabric. This phenomenon is due to the transformation of mechanical energy into heat by internal friction phenomena during the oscillations of the molecules. The interface is the surface that separates two tissues. These tissues have a different composition and elasticity that influences the speed of propagation of the wave.

The speed through the tissues is around 1540 m/second

FABRIC	ACOUSTIC IMPEDANCE (104/kg/m2/s)
Air	0,0004
Water	1,48
Blood	1,68
Reinetrate	1,62
Liver	1,63à1,67
Muscle	1,67à1,76
Bones	3,65à7

A fabric also has a resistance to the propagation of the wave is called the impedanceZ

Take home message

☐ The closer the tissue impedances are, the more the intensity reflected at the interface is low: In this case the wave will be mostly transmitted (eg liver / kidney interface)

☐ The more different the fabric impedances are, the more the wave undergoes a total reflection ex 'air/bone or liquid interface)

Hence the interest in using the gel between the probe and the skin to eliminate the film of air that can be interposed between the probe and the skin

Take home message

▪The acoustic impedance represents the resistance of the medium to the propagation of the wave

▪An acoustic interface is the separation surface between two tissues with different impedances

- The wave that comes into contact with an interface undergoes phenomena that will define the image obtained

- The greater the difference in impedance between the fabrics, the more the sound will be reflected rather than transmitted

- The Detection of echoes of return provides two pieces of information:

☐ Time taken by echo to reach the detector = depth of the interface
☐ Echo intensity depending on the size of the interface, i.e. the difference between the impedances of the adjacent media

Interaction phenomena

• Transmission and reflection The gel increases the transmission of waves between the probe and the tissues.

- Refraction:

- deviation of the transmitted beam when it is not perpendicular to the surface
- the deflection angle depends on the impedance

- Broadcasting:

- complex phenomenon of re-emission of a fraction of the wave in all directions
- occurs when the wave hits a structure smaller than the wave

- Mitigation:

- corresponds to the loss of energy of the acoustic wave when it meets tissues, which results in a decrease in its amplitude

The physical interactions between the waves and the media they encounter cause alterations in the image, which are called artifacts.

Types of probes

(Images from PHT 6011 - Advanced Cardiopulmonary Rehabilitation, U of M)

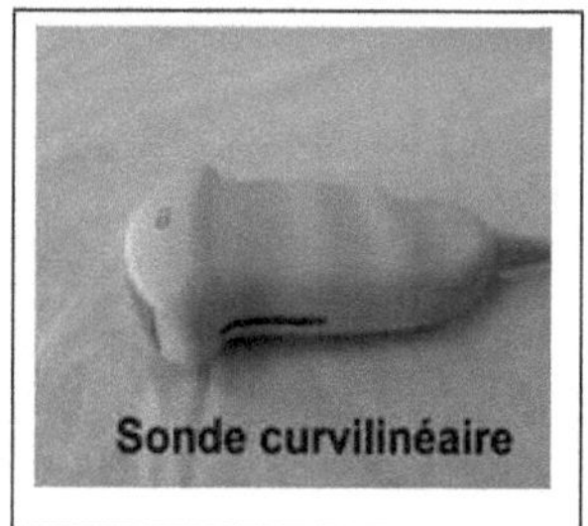

✓ **LINEAR**

High frequencies (7-18 MHz) for the examination of superficial structures

- Pleura

- Diaphragm attachment area (DAA)

- Larger footprint than the heart probe

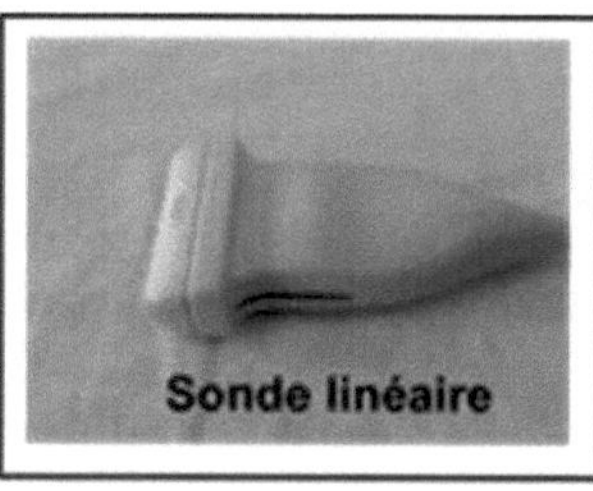

✓ **CURVILINEAR**

Low frequencies (3.5-5 MHz) for the examination of deep structures

- Alveolar-interstitial syndrome

- Pleural effusion

- Consolidation

- Curved footprint

✓ **CARDIAC (sectorial)**

Low frequencies (1.4-8 MHz) for the examination of deep structures

✓ Diaphragm

✓ Pleural space perdiaphragm

✓ No deformation of the structures

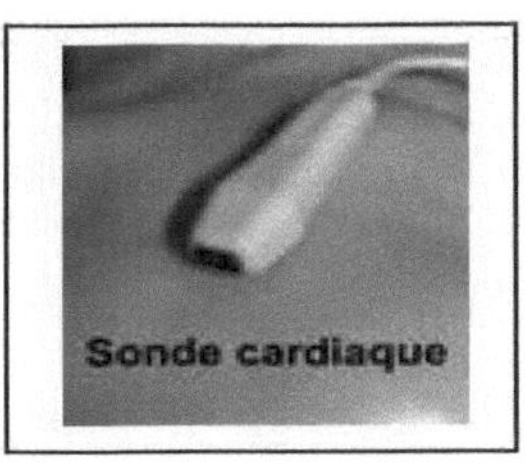

Echogeneity

Ability of a structure or interface to reflect ultrasound:

- hyperechoic structure forms a clear image

- structureisoechogenic forms a gray image

- anechoic structure forms a black image

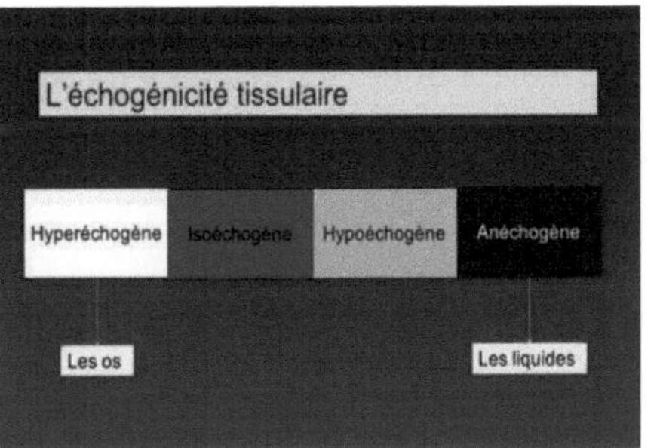

Image created by Stéphanie Grégoire, physiotherapist at the MHI

- OS: hyperechoic + pure shadow cone

- Water: anechoic + posterior reinforcement

- Air: hyperechoic + impure shadow cone

- Tissue: fat + echogenic than muscle, than liver

Different echogenicity visualized on the same image

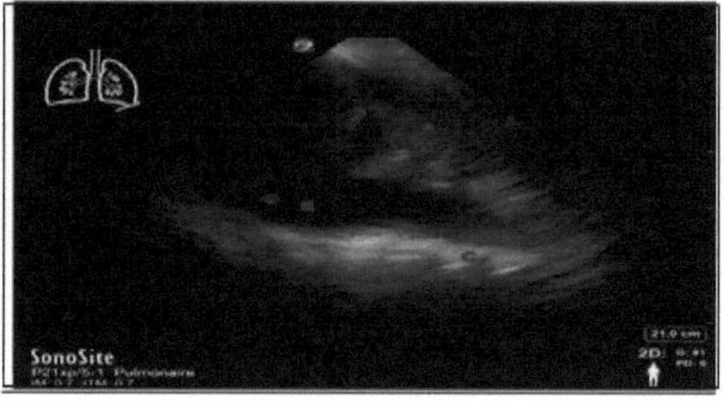

A.isoechogenic

B. anechoic

C.hyperechoic

Ultrasound image from Dr. André Denault's bank

CLASSIC AGREEMENT

On the screen, the marker is on the left:

- The patient's right is on the left of the screen (for a transverse axis)

- The patient's head is on the left of t h e   screen (for a longitudinal or sagittal axis)

- The top of the screen corresponds to the superficial structures (skin, near the probe)

- The bottom of the screen corresponds to the deep structures

Parameters

✓ **Depth:**

- analyzed by the delay between the transmission and reception of the wave

- adjusted to have structure studied in the center of the screen

✓ **Gain**

- adjusts the received signal strength to compensate for the attenuation

✓ **Focus**

- allows to improve the resolution of structures located at a desired depth

✓ **Scanning modes**

B Mode (Brilliance):

- Real-time, two-dimensional imaging

- Creation of an image using a combination of several ultrasound shots

M Mode (Time-Motion):

- - Juxtaposition of images recorded by a single shot in B-mode that shows the evolution of structures over time

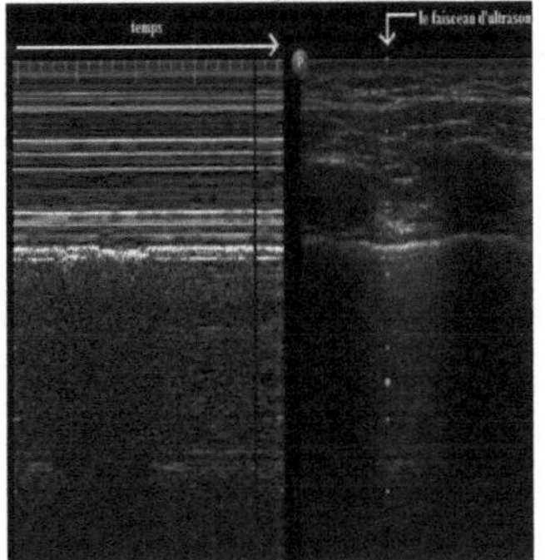

Ultrasound image from Dr. André Denault's bank

The Color Doppler mode applies a reference box to the resulting ultrasound image, in which you can see the color representing movement toward or away from the probe. This can be useful for identifying movement within a vessel to see if it is gaping.

The **blue** or **red** color represents the direction of flow, but does not determine whether the vessel is an artery or a vein.

Spectral or pulsed Doppler: provides a reference point that is applied to a vessel of interest, to hear and see changes in flow over time, as indicated by changes in the Doppler waveform. This mode is useful for determining whether a vessel is an artery or a vein, or for measuring the flow velocity through an opening, such as a heart valve, to determine the degree of stenosis.

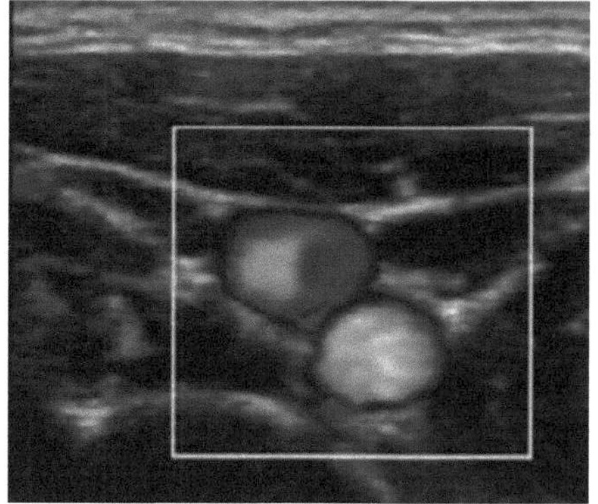

Figure. Color Doppler of vessels demonstrates active flows.

BAT sign "bat sign".

Since **several structures** as well as **the pleural line** may appear as a horizontal hyperechoic line (white) on the US screen, it is essential to be able to identify which of these lines represents the pleura. LICHTENSTEIN et al [ref:4. Lichtenstein DA, Pinsky R, Jardin F. General Ultrasound in the Critically Ill. Berlin, Springer, 2007] describes how to use the "bat sign" to facilitate correct identification of the pleural line.The term "bat sign" is used since the two ribs delineating an intercostal space (hyperechoic surface with posterior shadow cone) and the pleural line resembles a bat flying towards the screen (Figure). Thus, the following two steps:

1) make sure the scan plane is vertical and the orientation mark is at the top

2) use the "bat sign" as a sign to identify the pleural line.

Once this is done, the transducer can be rotated approximately 90° (depending on the angle of the ribs at the scanned area) counterclockwise to avoid the ribs and visualize the entire pleural line in the intercostal space.

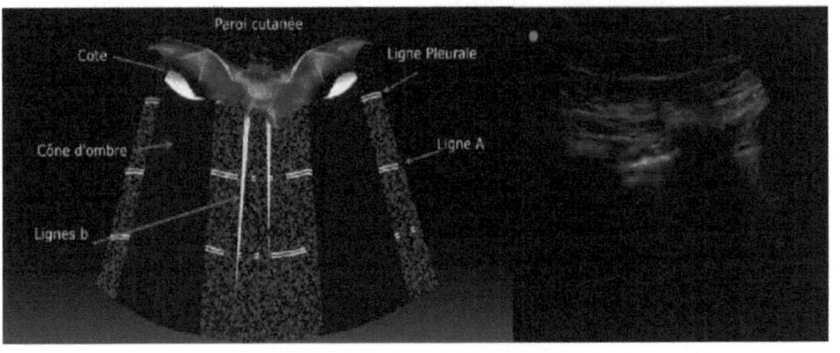

BAT sign or Bat sign

Thoracic wall: (muscles and fascias)

Corresponds to an alternation of horizontal lines, hypo- or hyperechoic, not mobile to respiratory movements.

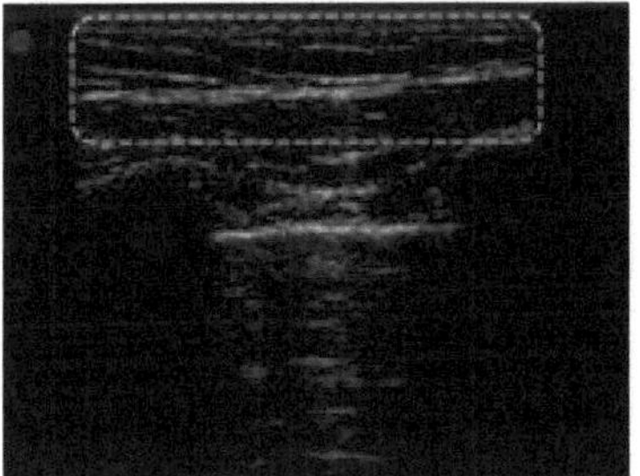

Costal arches (ribs):

Hyperechoic line, convex towards the wall, with a pure shadow cone

Intercostal space (or costo-intercostal):

Calculated from the top of the rib to the ventilated lung line, its thickness is 8 ± 2mm. It is pathological when it becomes greater than 10mm

Subpleural fatty border:

hypoechoic line less than 2 mm thick, sub pleural, just before the lung, independent of respiratory movements

Pleural line:

It is a hyperechoic, regular, continuous line with an impure shadow cone. It can be the site of an interruption of less than 1mm with a maximum of 3 interruptions per field.

Lung artifacts:

Reverberation artifacts: A lines

Reverberation occurs when the emitted beam bounces back and forth between two reflective Interfaces.This may appear as recurring bright hyperechogenic lines at equidistant intervals from the transducer at the bottom of the screen. These reflections between the transducer and the pleura generate "A-lines" (Figure 1). A distance equal to the initial index distance between the skin and the pleura separates the sequential artifact lines.

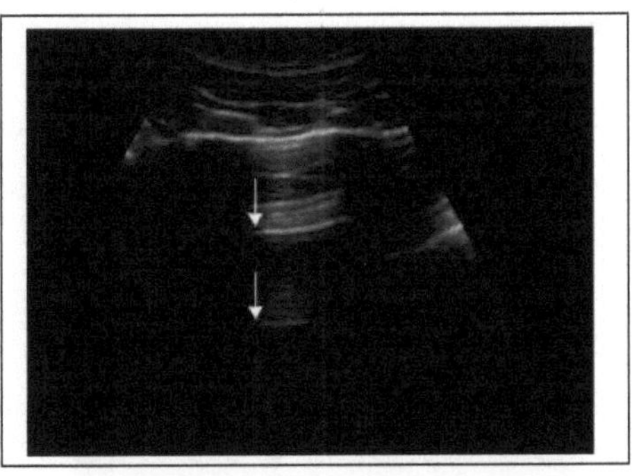

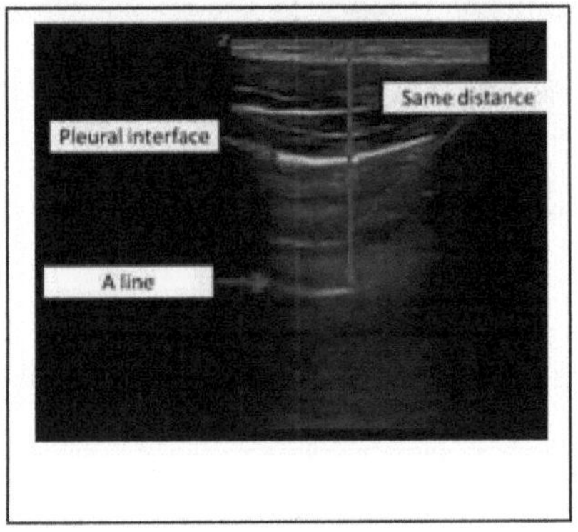

Figure: Reverberation artifacts, known as A-lines (arrows), extending to the bottom of the screen, spaced at equidistant intervals from each other.

Ultrasound characteristics of the A lines

☐ Horizontal line, hyperechoic

☐ Each A-line is located at a distance from the probe that is a multiple of the distance between the probe and the pleura

☐ A deep A-line cannot exist without a larger A-line

Refraction artifacts: B lines

A refraction artifact occurs when an emitted sound beam passes through surfaces of different densities at an oblique angle. An acoustic shadow will appear posterior to the point at which the beam crossed this tissue interface and changed direction.

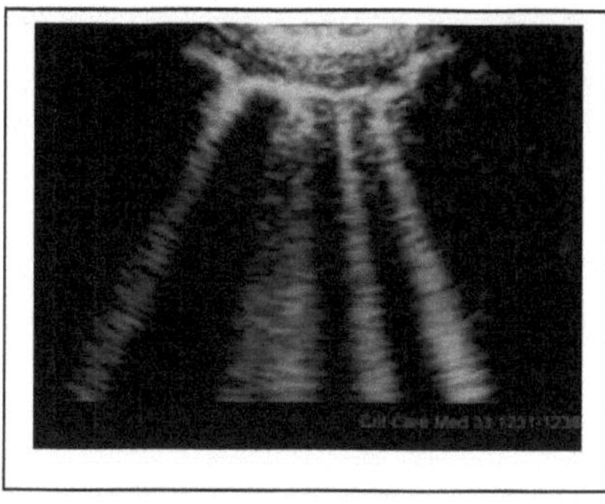

Line B comet tail artifacts

arghetta R. J. Clin. Ultrasound, 1993

Ultrasound characteristics

- Hyper-echogenic vertical line, well defined
- Origin of the pleural line
- Crosses the screen to the depth of the comet tail
- Deletes all other images on its path (e.g., line A)
- Moves with pleural slip (if pleural origin)

Assessment of the pleural line

The presence or absence of these signs is important when evaluating the pleural line and the underlying lung:

1) **pleural slip,**

2) **line(s) B.**

3) Sign of the shore

4) pulmonary pulse

The pleural slip

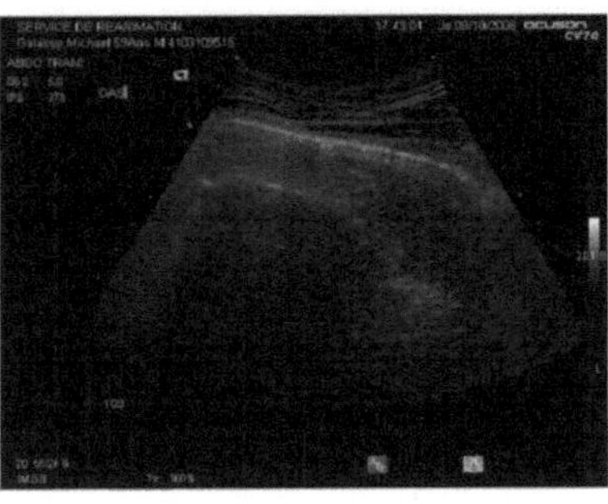

Pleural slip is seen, **in B-mode,** as a horizontal movement of the pleural line in synchrony with the respiratory cycle, indicating a sliding movement of the visceral pleura against the parietal pleura [3, 5].

Pleural slippage is due to the up and down movement of the visceral pleura in synchrony with the piston-like respiratory movements of the diaphragm [6].

When air separates the two pleural sheets (in case of pneumothorax, the movement disappears and cannot be detected by US. In such a case, the pleural line represents only the parietal pleura, which is still visible but not slippery since it is attached to the chest wall [5, 9].

Apart from pneumothorax, other pathologies can also cause the absence of pleural slip (e.g. pulmonary fibrosis, purulent pleurisy or operative sequelae of thoracic surgery) [6-8, 10, 11].

B lines

A B-line has been defined as a laser-like hyperechoic vertical reverberation artifact arising from the pleural line. B-lines are continuous from the pleural line to the bottom edge of the screen and do not fade [3, 13, 14]. Other reverberation artifacts may also originate from the pleural line, but unlike the B-lines, they fade relatively quickly and do not continue to the lower edge of the screen (Figure 4) [3, 4]. If pleural slip is present, the B-lines move in synchrony with the slip [15].

Shoreline Sign:

The shore sign (or seaside sign) is defined in TM mode. It corresponds to the sub pleural lung movements. The resulting cloud of points under the pleural line draws the image corresponding to the shoreline sign. The presence of the latter in TM mode confirms the lung's adherence to the wall and the absence of a pneumothorax.

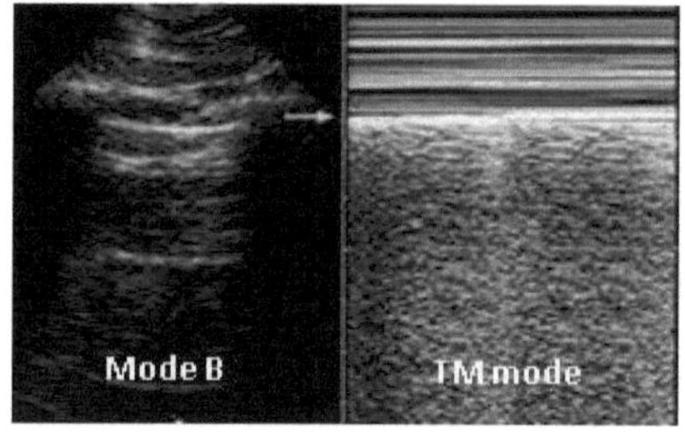

Pulmonary pulse:

In addition to pleural sliding in synchrony with the respiratory cycle, the pleural line and underlying lung can also move in synchrony with **the heartbeat**. This movement, called the "pulmonary pulse," is caused by the force of the heartbeat transmitted to the lung and thus to the visceral pleura [3, 7]. The pulmonary pulse is best visualized in time-motion (TM) mode and its presence indicates the presence of the lung. The pulmonary pulse is not always present in healthy individuals and is generally easier to visualize in areas where the lung is in close contact with the pericardium and heart. Like pleural slip, the pulmonary pulse indicates that the lung, viscera, and parietal pleural surfaces are juxtaposed at the probe site [7, 8, 12].

Several factors can affect the magnitude of the pulmonary pulse (e.g., lung area scanned, patient tidal volume, underlying pulmonary pathology, and intubation) [6-8].

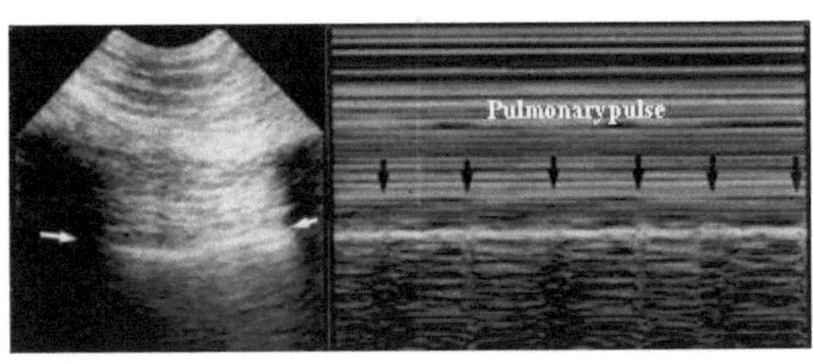

Take home message

The hyperechoic horizontal line with impure shadow cone corresponds to the pleuropulmonary line if: In B mode:

- There are B lines

- There is a pleural slip In TM mode:

- There is a sign of the shore

- There is a pulmonary pulse

Diaphragm and adjacent abdominal structures

Recognition and identification of the diaphragm and abdominal structures is an essential part of the FTUS and TUS, as these structures serve as important anatomical landmarks to differentiate intra-thoracic structures from abdominal structures.

Diaphragm

The superficial part of the diaphragm can be recognized as a hyperechoic "double line" located just below the ribs and is best seen subcostally through the spleen by the high frequency linear probe. The most hypoechoic area between the lines represents the muscle fibers of the diaphragm. As the diaphragm contracts, the movement and thickening of the fibers can be observed [17]. The most central part or tendon component of the diaphragm can be visualized when using the liver or spleen as an acoustic window [18-21].

During the movements of respiration, and in the absence of an obstacle between the lung and the diaphragm, the impure shadow cone of the aerated lung comes to cover the diaphragm and the underlying structures with each inspiration like a curtain. This sign is called **the thoracoabdominal junction sign or the curtain sign.** Diaphragmatic stroke, or diaphragmatic excursion, is measured in TM mode, and is the distance the diaphragm travels between inspiration and expiration. The normal range of diaphragmatic stroke is usually greater than 2.5cm with a difference of less than 50% between the two sides.

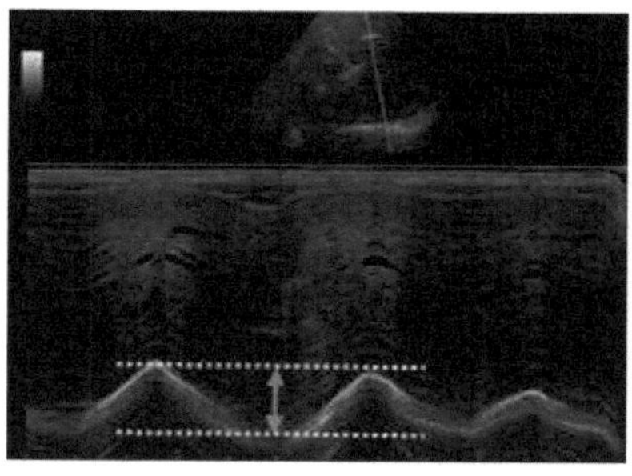

Focused TUS

The purpose of FTUS is most often to diagnose or exclude acute, life-threatening disease [22].When performing FTUS, usually only a limited area of the pleural and lung surface is evaluated, and it can therefore be performed quickly with minimal discomfort to the critically ill patient [24, 25]. The use of FTUS has been shown to have a diagnostic accuracy effect for many common conditions seen in a variety of emergencies [3, 10, 24, 26-34]. When used as part of a whole body ultrasound,FTUS has been shown to help identify patients with undetected life-threatening conditions and has significantly increased the proportion of patients correctly diagnosed and treated in the emergency department with respiratory symptoms [35, 36].

FTUS, along with other forms of targeted US, should be used as an integral part of the clinical evaluation of these patients.

FTUS Scanning Protocols

Several different FTUS protocols and approaches have been described; however, An international consensus for the use of a specific protocol has been reached[3]. The protocols divide the chest into a number of scan areas that are Evaluated by ultrasound. [4, 9, 12,13, 31, 37-48].

The number of scanned areas is important for the diagnosis. The criteria for certain conditions (e.g. interstitial syndrome) are defined by the number of areas in which specific results are represented.In this way, the number of zones can potentially affect the accuracy of diagnosis compared to other protocols or use in other settings [3, 24, 31, 49].

In addition to protocols describing FTUS, several other studies have described the use of FTUS principles as an integral part of a whole-body ultrasound approach in which multiple organs or structures are assessed in the clinical setting [4, 34, 35, 50- 54]. Many studies have used an eight-scan-zone approach, as described by VOLPICELLI et al [44], to evaluate anterior and lateral thoracic surfaces. (However, this approach does not include evaluation of the posterior thoracic region, so posteriorly positioned pathology may be missed using this protocol [44 LAURSEN et al [35] modified the 14-zone protocol (fig below) by adding assessment of the posterior surfaces using the same principles originally described by LICHTENSTEIN et al [4], prospective studies in various settings [35, 36, 55, 56]. The use of this 14-zone FTUS approach in parallel with FoCUS has been validated to assess patients with respiratory failure in an emergency department [35, 36].

Using the 14-zone approach, each hemithorax is divided into anterior, lateral, and posterior surfaces, which can be subdivided into small squares representing a scan zone. Each of these scan zones should be assessed using FTUS. Each of the scan areas can be scored from 1R to 7R on the right and 1L to 7L on the left (Figure 5) [35]. As described in the following sections, when evaluating the As described in the following sections, when assessing the lateral and posterior surface, it is essential to begin the assessment by identifying the upper abdominal structures and the diaphragm. This is done to avoid confusing abdominal structures with thoracic structures and vice versa (e.g., stomach misdiagnosed as pleural effusion). To facilitate this approach, caudal areas (e.g., areas 3 and 5) have smaller numbers than cranial areas (e.g., areas 4, 6, and 7) [35].

Terms such as "normal review" should generally be negated as they imply TUS performance.

FTUS reports were limited to answering the questions: "No evidence of PTX, pleural effusion or interstitial syndrome.

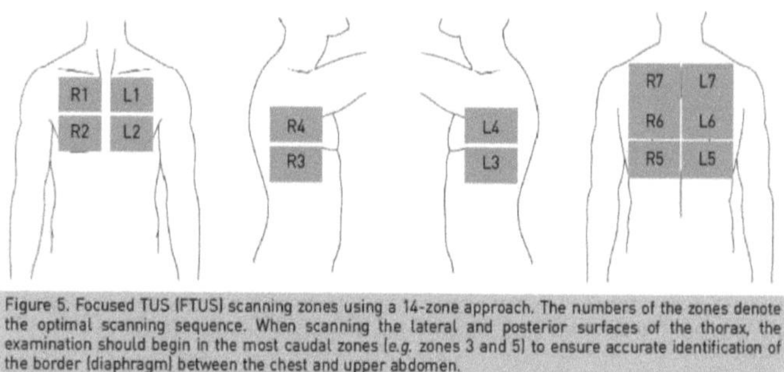

Figure 5. Focused TUS (FTUS) scanning zones using a 14-zone approach. The numbers of the zones denote the optimal scanning sequence. When scanning the lateral and posterior surfaces of the thorax, the examination should begin in the most caudal zones (e.g. zones 3 and 5) to ensure accurate identification of the border (diaphragm) between the chest and upper abdomen.

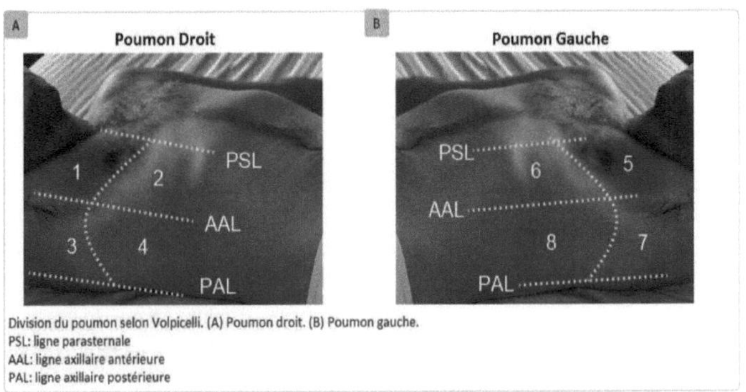

Volpicelli G, et al. Intensive Care Med. 2012;38(4):577-91

Image from and adapted from: Basic Transesophageal and Critical Care Ultrasound, Taylor and Francis, CRC Press, 2016, p. 249

Synthesis

SIGN OR ARTIFACT	MODE B
Pleural line	x
Sign of the bat	x
Shading	x
Pleural slippage	x
Sign of the beach	
A lines	x
B lines	x

Pathological aspects:

✓ **Pleural effusion**

The role of thoracic ultrasound is:

- **Estimate the volume of the effusion**

- **Identify the type of pleural effusion**

- **To guide a pleural gesture**

Pleural fluid effusion is usually visualized by using a low-frequency convex probe in B mode.The first step in exploring for pleurisy is positioning the patient. Generally, the patient should be seated, the operator locates the diaphragm and moves up the thorax to explore the pleural effusion. The pleural fluid effusion presents on ultrasound as an **anechoic image with posterior enhancement.**

The appearance of the effusion may vary depending on the nature of the fluid, it may be :
- Anechoic

- Echogen

- Heterogeneous

- Free

- Partitioned

• **The image of a transudate is perfectly black (always anechoic)**

• **The image of an exudate may be anechoic or echogenic**

• **Empyema and hemothorax usually present as an echogenic and heterogeneous image.**

• **An echogenic, heterogeneous or compartmentalized appearance always points to an exudate.**

Fig free anechoic pleurisy Fig compartmentalized pleurisy

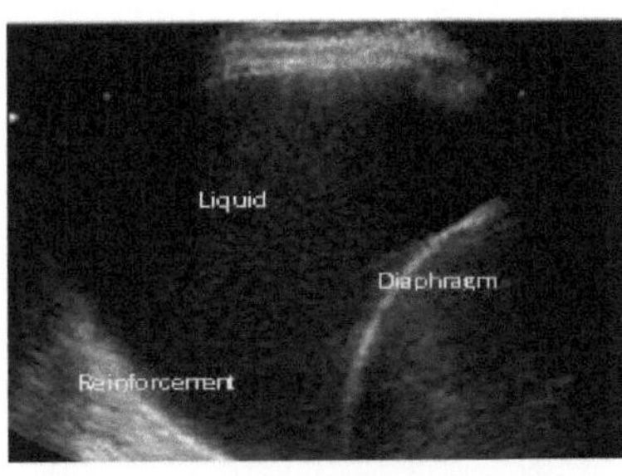

**Aspect of an exudate with echogenic appearance of the fluid
(https://splf.fr/wp- content/uploads/2014/12/Echography-in-pleural-
pathology-CPLF-2015-Gilles- Mangiapan.pdf)**

Pneumothorax

Sensitivity: 88%.

Specificity: 99%.

Ultrasound criteria:

A pneumothorax is best visualized with a high-frequency linear probe in longitudinal and intercostal sections.

A pneumothorax on ultrasound is characterized by:

- The absence of a pleural slip in B mode.

- The absence of B lines in B mode

- The absence of the shoreline sign in TM mode, which is replaced by a barcode sign.

- Absence of the pulmonary pulse in TM mode.

- The presence of the lung point or the point of attachment: which means the point of attachment of the lung to the wall in the presence of a partial pneumothorax. It is the transition point between the barcode sign and the shoreline sign in TM mode.

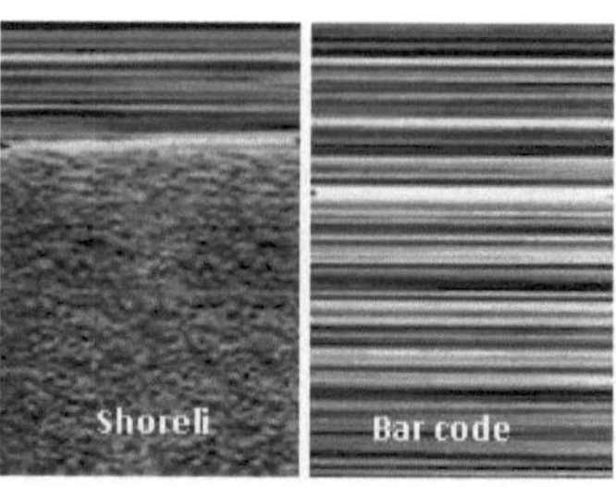

Fig: Bar code sign (indicating the presence of a pneumothorax)

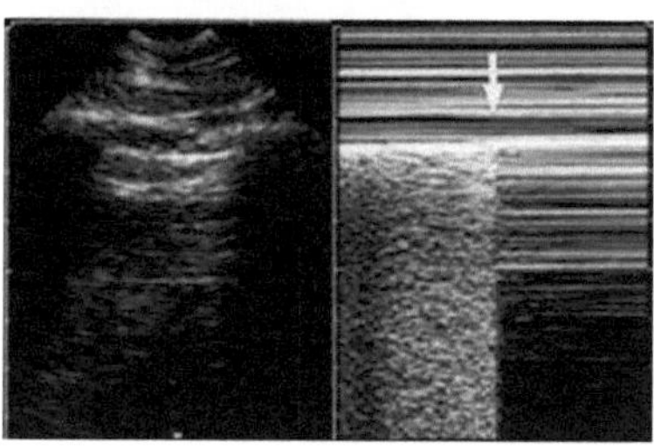

Fig: lung point (https://www.srlf.org/wp- content/uploads/2015/11/0301-Reanimation-Vol12-N1-p019_029.pdf)

✓ **Signs of exclusion of pneumothorax:**

- **Pleural slippage**

- **"Lung pulse**

- **Presence of one or more B lines**

ADVANTAGES AND LIMITATIONS of ultrasound as a means of exploring the thorax Practical and allowing a rapid evaluation in real time, US also has the advantage of being able to be coupled with a diagnostic procedure.38 It is recommended before all pleural procedures to limit complications and improve diagnostic yield.39-41 Compared with CT-scan-guided biopsies, the occurrence of bleeding complications is comparable in US. There are fewer pneumothoraxes and the intervention time is shorter under US.42,43 It is at least as effective as CT-scan for the diagnosis of peripheral or parietal lung lesions by biopsy, at a lower cost and without exposure to radiation.44,45 The characteristics of the wall may limit exploration (obesity, dressing, chest drain, subcutaneous emphysema, osteosynthesis material, extensive pleural calcification). Without pleural contact, the more central pathologies escape transthoracic US. Concerning the ultrasound evaluation of the diaphragm, it is less good than fluoroscopy, in particular for the analysis of the kinetics (interposition of the intestines, air bubble g

Step-by-step approach

1. Place the linear probe over the anterior thorax, at the level of the first intercostal space of the medioclavicular line in which you can identify the pleural line between two ribs.
2. The marker should be pointed at the patient's head in the sagittal plane.

3. Look for the pleural interface that is bordered by the rib shadow. Center the image between two intercostal spaces.
4. Look for pleural slippage during breathing. This will look like a line of ants along the pleural interface.
5. Look for comet tail artifacts corresponding to the B lines.

6. If no pleural slip is observed or if the case is difficult to examine, use M mode to look for signs of the seaside or stratosphere.
7. Repeat steps 3-6 on three additional intercostal spaces for each side.

8. If pneumothorax is suspected, place the patient on oxygen, consider a chest x-ray and placement of a chest tube.

9. If a pleural effusion is observed, an ultrasound-guided pleural puncture may be performed.

Interest of thoracic ultrasound in medical thoracoscopy:

Clinical case:

A 71-year-old female patient with a history of coronary artery disease and medical therapy was presented with progressively worsening dyspnea over several weeks, revealing the presence of a large fluid pleural effusion.

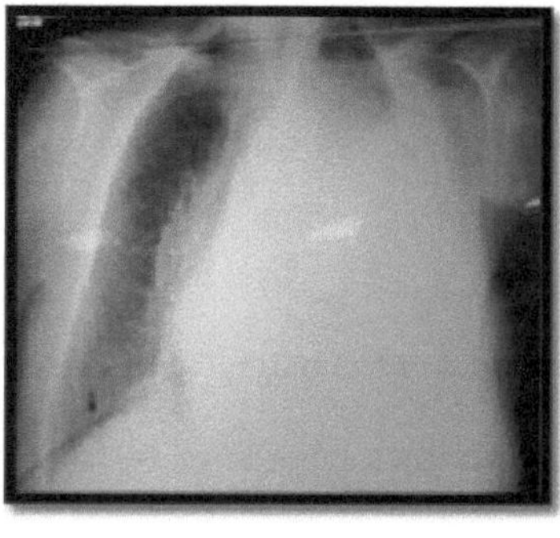

Fig: Frontal chest radiograph showing the presence of a watery opacity that occupies the lower two-thirds of the left lung field, obliterating the diaphragmatic dome and filling the pleural sacs with an upper limit concave upward and inward toward the lung parenchyma with a mediastinal deviation on the contralateral side, suggesting a pleurisy of great abundance

A blind pleural puncture after clinical examination was attempted with failure to locate the fluid. A pleural ultrasound was performed, showing the presence of an irregular thickening of the pleura with a deep localization of the pleural fluid. Hence the importance of the thoracic ultrasound, which made it possible to rule out the presence of a pneumothorax that could complicate the pleural puncture, and to carry out various measurements in order to be able to choose a needle of adequate size and guide the pleural puncture in complete safety.

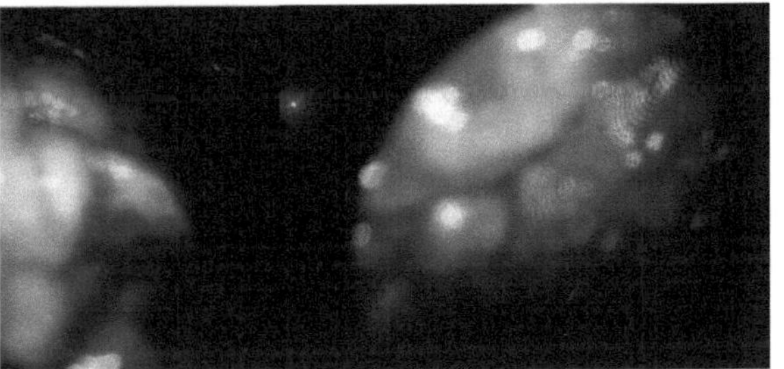

Fig: A: Chest ultrasound showing irregular pleural thickening with anechoic pleural fluid. B: Measurement of the depth of the effusion and the thickness of the pleura.

The patient underwent medical thoracoscopy for diagnostic and therapeutic purposes to better characterize the pleural appearance, to direct pleural biopsies, to drain the pleural effusion and to perform pleurodesis to prevent recurrence of the effusion.

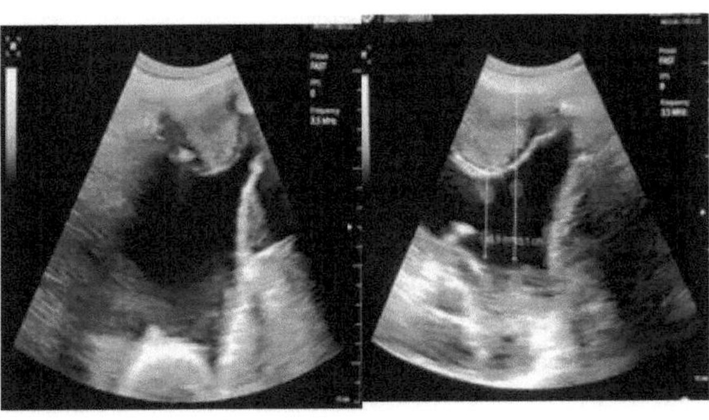

Fig: Thoracoscopic appearance of medical pleuroscopy under local anesthesia showing the irregular and multinodular appearance of the pleura.

A thoracoscopically guided biopsy of the nodules was performed, and pathological and immunohistochemical examination concluded that the localization pleural extramedullary plasmacytoma or multiple plasmacytomas with a pleural localization.

Contribution of thoracic ultrasound in medical pleuroscopy:

The interest of thoracic ultrasound in medical thoracoscopy is multiple:

Before pleuroscopy: Ultrasound allows to :

➢ **Check for the presence of pleural fluid and its abundance.**

➢ **Study the appearance of the liquid (free or partitioned).**

➢ **Evaluate the pleura (presence of adhesions, pachypleuritis, nodules...)**

➢ **Check the vascularity using the Doppler mode.**

➢ **Decrease multiple radiations due to standard radiography and CT scan.**

During pleuroscopy:

➢ **Orient the front door safely.**

After the procedure is completed:

➢ **Check for a pneumothorax complicating the procedure (look for pleural shift and B-lines in B-mode, and pulmonary pulse and shore sign in M-mode).**

➢ **Follow the evolution of the pleural effusion (recurrence?)**

➢ **Reduce the need for surgery.**

ANNEXES

BLUE PROTOCOL

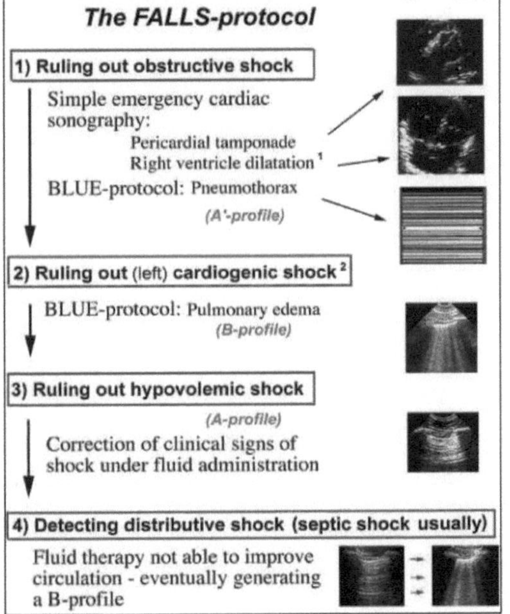

Arbre décisionnel du **BLUE-Protocol** selon Lichtenstein

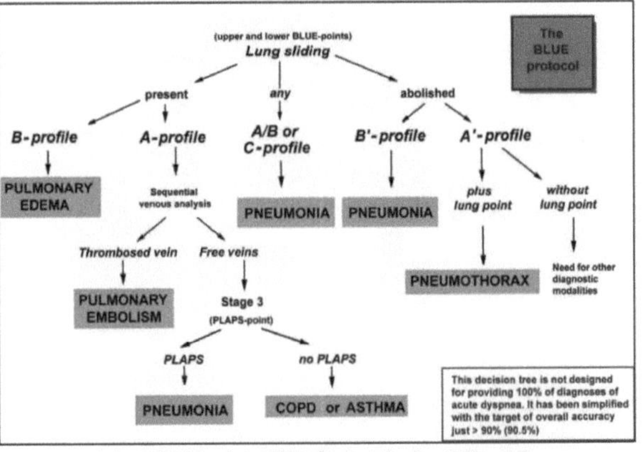

Arbre décisionnel du **FALLS**-Protocol

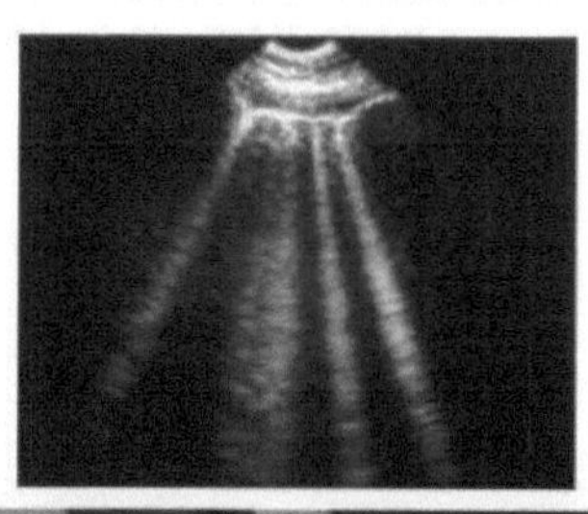

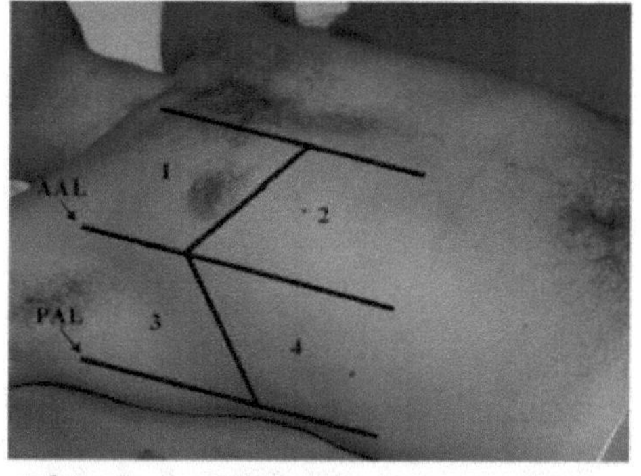

Méthode de Volpicelli : diagnostic d'œdème interstitiel posé si présence d'au moins 2 lignes B dans une de ces 4 zones de façon bilatérale

REFERENCES

1. Norman W.RantanenDVM, MS1The use of diagnostic ultrasound in limb disorders of the horse: A preliminary report Journal of Equine Veterinary Science Volume 2, Issue 2, 1982, Pages 62-

2. Moore CL, Copel JA. Point-of-care ultrasonography. The New England journal of medicine 2011; 364: 749-57.

3. Noble VE, Nelson BP. Manual of Emergency and Critical Care Ultrasound: Cambridge University Press, 2011.

4. Via G, Hussain A, Wells M, Reardon R, ElBarbary M, Noble VE, Tsung JW, Neskovic AN, Price S, Oren-Grinberg A, Liteplo A, Cordioli R, Naqvi N, Rola P, Poelaert J, Guliĉ TG, Sloth E, Labovitz A, Kimura B, Breitkreutz R, Masani N, Bowra J, Talmor D, Guarracino F, Goudie A, Xiaoting W, Chawla R, Galderisi M27, Blaivas M, Petrovic T, Storti E, Neri L, Melniker L; International Liaison Committee on Focused Cardiac UltraSound (ILC-FoCUS); International Conference on Focused Cardiac UltraSound (IC-FoCUS). International evidence-based recommendations for focused cardiac ultrasound. J Am Soc Echocardiogr. 2014 Jul;27(7):683.e1-683.e33. doi: 10.1016/j.echo.2014.05.001.

5. Volpicelli G, Elbarbary M, Blaivas M, Lichtenstein DA, Mathis G, Kirkpatrick AW, Melniker L, Gargani L, Noble VE, Via G, Dean A, Tsung JW, Soldati G, Copetti R, Bouhemad B, Reissig A, Agricola E, Rouby JJ, Arbelot C, Liteplo A, Sargsyan A, Silva F, Hoppmann R, Breitkreutz R, Seibel A, Neri L, Storti E, Petrovic T, International Liaison Committee on Lung Ultrasound for International Consensus Conference on Lung U. International evidence-based recommendations for point-of-care lung ultrasound. Intensive care medicine2012; 38: 577-91.

6. 23. Rumack CM, Wilson SR, Charboneau JW, et al. Diagnostic Ultrasound. 4th Edn. St Louis, Elsevier/Mosby, 2011.

7. 24. Lichtenstein DA, Meziere GA. Relevance of lung ultrasound in the diagnosis of acute respiratory failure: the BLUE

8. protocol. Chest 2008; 134: 117-125.

9. 25. Laursen CB, Sloth E, Lassen AT, et al. Does point-of-care ultrasonography cause discomfort in patients admitted

10. with respiratory symptoms? Scand J Trauma Resusc Emerg Med 2015; 23: 46.

11. 26. Squizzato A, Rancan E, Dentali F, et al. Diagnostic accuracy of lung ultrasound for pulmonary embolism: a

12. systematic review and meta-analysis. J Thromb Haemost 2013; 11: 1269-1278.

13. 27. Chavez MA, Shams N, Ellington LE, et al. Lung ultrasound for the diagnosis of pneumonia in adults: a systematic

14. review and meta-analysis. Respir Res 2014; 15: 50.

15. 28. Al Deeb M, Barbic S, Featherstone R, et al. Point-of-care ultrasonography for the diagnosis of acute cardiogenic

16. pulmonary edema in patients presenting with acute dyspnea: a systematic review and meta-analysis. Acad Emerg

17. Med 2014; 21: 843-852.

18. 29. Pivetta E, Goffi A, Lupia E, et al. Lung ultrasound-implemented diagnosis of acute decompensated heart failure in

19. the ED: a SIMEU multicenter study. Chest 2015; 148: 202-210.

20. 30. Rempell JS, Noble VE. Using lung ultrasound to differentiate patients in acute dyspnea in the prehospital

21. emergency setting. Crit Care 2011; 15: 161.

22. 31. Laursen CB, Hänselmann A, Posth S, et al. Prehospital lung ultrasound for the diagnosis of cardiogenic pulmonary

23. Oedema: a pilot study. Scand J Trauma Resusc Emerg Med 2016; 24: 96.

24. 32. Neesse A, Jerrentrup A, Hoffmann S, et al. Prehospital chest emergency sonography trial in Germany: a

25. prospective study. Eur J Emerg Med 2012; 19: 161-166.

26. 33. Kristensen MS, Teoh WH, Graumann O, et al. Ultrasonography for clinical decision-making and intervention in

27. Airway management: from the mouth to the lungs and pleurae. Insights Imaging 2014; 5: 253-279.

28. 34. Kirkpatrick AW, Sirois M, Laupland KB, et al. Hand-held thoracic sonography for detecting post-traumatic

29. pneumothoraces: the Extended Focused Assessment with Sonography for Trauma (EFAST). J Trauma 2004; 57: 288-295.

30. 35. Laursen CB, Sloth E, Lambrechtsen J, et al. Focused sonography of the heart, lungs, and deep veins identifies

31. missed life-threatening conditions in admitted patients with acute respiratory symptoms. Chest 2013; 144: 1868- 1875.

32. 36. Laursen CB, Sloth E, Lassen AT, et al. Point-of-care ultrasonography in patients admitted with respiratory

33. symptoms: a single-blind, randomised controlled trial. Lancet Respir Med 2014; 2: 638-646.

34. 37. Targhetta R, Chavagneux R, Bourgeois JM, et al. Sonographic approach to diagnosing pulmonary consolidation.

35. J Ultrasound Med 1992; 11: 667-672.

36. 38. Reissig A, Kroegel C. Transthoracic sonography of diffuse parenchymal lung disease: the role of comet tail artifacts.

37. J Ultrasound Med 2003; 22: 173-180.

38. Jambrik Z, Monti S, Coppola V, et al. Usefulness of ultrasound lung comets as a nonradiologic sign ofextravascular lung water. Am J Cardiol 2004; 93: 1265-1270.

39. 40. Agricola E, Bove T, Oppizzi M, et al. "Ultrasound comet-tail images: a marker of pulmonary edema: a

40. comparative study with wedge pressure and extravascular lung water. Chest 2005; 127: 1690-1695.

41. 41. Bedetti G, Gargani L, Corbisiero A, et al. Evaluation of ultrasound lung comets by hand-held echocardiography.

42. Cardiovasc Ultrasound 2006; 4: 34.

43. 42. Picano E, Frassi F, Agricola E, et al. Ultrasound lung comets: a clinically useful sign of extravascular lung water.

44. J Am Soc Echocardiogr 2006; 19: 356-363.

45. 43. Soldati G, Testa A, Silva FR, et al. Chest ultrasonography in lung contusion. Chest 2006; 130: 533-538.

46. 44. Volpicelli G, Mussa A, Garofalo G, et al. Bedside lung ultrasound in the assessment of alveolar-interstitial

47. syndrome. Am J Emerg Med 2006; 24: 689-696.

48. 45. Fagenholz PJ, Gutman JA, Murray AF, et al. Chest ultrasonography for the diagnosis and monitoring of

49. high-altitude pulmonary edema. Chest 2007; 131: 1013-1018.

50. 46. Bouhemad B, Liu ZH, Arbelot C, et al. Ultrasound assessment of antibiotic- induced pulmonary reaeration in

51. ventilator-associated pneumonia. Crit Care Med 2010; 38: 84-92.

52. 47. Via G, Lichtenstein D, Mojoli F, et al. Whole lung lavage: a unique model for ultrasound assessment of lung

53. aeration changes. Intensive Care Med 2010; 36: 999-1007.

54. 48. Stefanidis K, Dimopoulos S, Kolofousi C, et al. Sonographic lobe localization of alveolar-interstitial syndrome in

55. Crit Care Res Pract 2012; 2012: 179719.

56. 49. Volpicelli G, Noble VE, Liteplo A, et al. Decreased sensitivity of lung ultrasound limited to the anterior chest in

57. emergency department diagnosis of cardiogenic pulmonary edema: a retrospective analysis. Crit Ultrasound J 2010;

58. 2: 47-52.

59. 50. Jensen MB, Sloth E, Larsen KM, et al. Transthoracic echocardiography for cardiopulmonary monitoring in

60. intensive care. Eur J Anaesthesiol 2004; 21: 700-707.

61. 51. Perera P, Mailhot T, Riley D, et al. The RUSH exam: Rapid Ultrasound in SHock in the evaluation of the critically

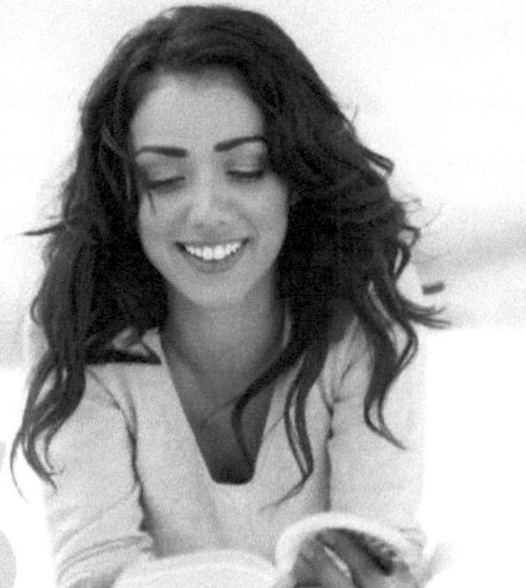

yes I want morebooks!

Buy your books fast and straightforward online - at one of world's fastest growing online book stores! Environmentally sound due to Print-on-Demand technologies.

Buy your books online at
www.morebooks.shop

Kaufen Sie Ihre Bücher schnell und unkompliziert online – auf einer der am schnellsten wachsenden Buchhandelsplattformen weltweit! Dank Print-On-Demand umwelt- und ressourcenschonend produziert.

Bücher schneller online kaufen
www.morebooks.shop

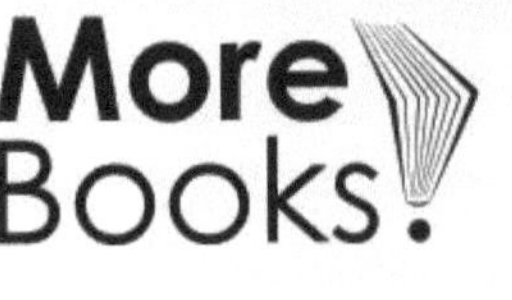

info@omniscriptum.com
www.omniscriptum.com

OMNIScriptum

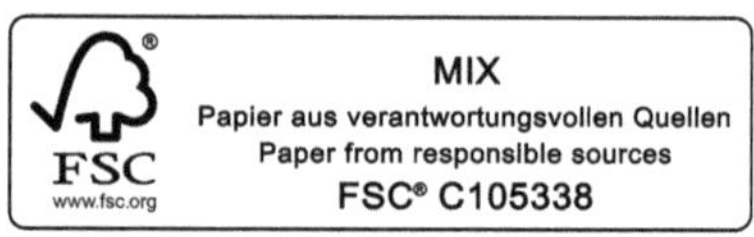

Printed by Books on Demand GmbH, Norderstedt / Germany